AF783748

Practical Manual of

PHARMACOLOGY AND TOXICOLOGY

For

Second Year Diploma Pharmacy Students

(According to PCI, ER 1991)

DR. G. D. GUPTA (M. Pharm. Ph. D, MBA)
DIRECTOR-CUM-PRINCIPAL
ISF COLLEGE OF PHARMACY, MOGA, PUNJAB.

DR. SHAILESH SHARMA (M. Pharm. Ph. D.)
PRINCIPAL
ASBASJSM DIPLOMA COLLEGE OF PHARMACY, BELA (ROPAR) PUNJAB.

HARSIMRAN SINGH (M. Pharm.)
ASSISTANT PROFESSOR (PHARMACOLOGY)
ASBASJSM COLLEGE OF PHARMACY, BELA (ROPAR) PUNJAB.

Name:____________________

Roll No.:____________________

Session:____________________

College Name:____________________

NIRALI PRAKASHAN
ADVANCEMENT OF KNOWLEDGE

N2588

PHARMACOLOGY AND TOXICOLOGY ISBN 978-93-86700-15-5

Fifth Edition : **February 2020**

Published By :

NIRALI PRAKASHAN

Abhyudaya Pragati, 1312, Shivaji Nagar
Off J.M. Road, PUNE – 411005
Tel - (020) 25512336/37/39, Fax - (020) 25511379
Email : niralipune@pragationline.com

CERTIFICATE

This is to certify that Mr. /Ms. ________________________________

is a regular student of ____

D. Pharmacy Second Year. He/She has completed his/her practical work of Pharmacology and Toxicology in the supervision of Dr./Mr./Ms. ______________ during the academic session 201__/201____.

Number of practicals performed ________ out of ________ in the subject of Pharmacology and Toxicology.

Roll No. _______________

Date:____/_____/________

Signature of Student

Teacher In-charge

Principal Signature

Institute Rubber Stamp

Syllabus ...

THEORY **(75 Hours)**

1. Introduction to Pharmacology, scope of Pharmacology.
2. Routes of administration of drugs, their advantages and disadvantages.
3. Various processes of absorption of drugs and the factors affecting them, Metabolism, distribution and excretion of drugs.
4. General mechanism of drugs action and the factors which modify drug action.
5. Pharmacological classification of drugs. The discussion of drugs should emphasize the following aspects:
   (i) Drugs acting on the Central Nervous System:
      (a) General anaesthetics, adjunction to anaesthesia, intravenous anasesthetics.
      (b) Analgesic antipyretics and non-steroidal anti-inflammatory drugs, Narcotic analgesics, Antirheumatic and antigout remedies, Sedatives and Hypnotics, Psychopharmacological agents, anticonvulsants, analeptics.
      (c) Centrally acting muscle relaxants and anti parkinsonism agents
   (ii) Local anaesthetics.
   (iii) Drug acting on autonomic nervous system.
      (a) Cholinergic drug, Anticholinergic drugs, anti cholinesterase drugs.
      (b) Adrenergic drugs and adrenergic recepter blockers.
      (c) Neurones blockers and ganglion blockers.
      (d) Neuromuscular blockers, drugs used in myasthenia gravis.
   (iv) Drugs acting on eye, mydriatics, drugs used in glaucoma.
   (v) Drugs acting on respiratory system-Respiratory stimulants, Bronchodilators, Nasal decongestants, Expectorants and Antitussive agents.
   (vi) Antacids, Physiological role of histamine and serotonin, Histamine and Antihistamines, Prostaglandins.
   (vii) Cardiovascular drugs, Cardiotonics, Antiarrhythmic agents, Antianginal agents, Antihypertensive agents, Peripheral Vasodilators and drugs used in atherosclerosis.
   (viii) Drugs acting on the blood and blood forming organs. Haematinics, Coagulants and Anticoagulants, Haemostatics, Blood substitutes and plasma expanders.
   (ix) Drugs affecting renal function - Diuretics and antidiuretics.
   (x) Hormones and hormone antagonists-hypoglycemic agents, Antithyroid drugs, sex hormones and oral contraceptives, corticosteroids.
   (xi) Drugs acting on digestive system - Carminatives, digestants Bitters, Antacids and drugs used in Peptic ulcer, purgatives, and laxatives, Antidiarrhoeals, Emetics, Antiemetics, Anti-spasmodics.
   Chemotherapy of microbial disease ;Urinary antiseptics, Sulphonamides, Penicillins, Streptomycin, Tetracylines and other antibiotics, Antitubercular agents, Antifungal agents, antiviral drugs, antileprotic drugs.
6. Chemotherapy of protozoal diseases Anthelmintic drugs.
7. Chemotherapy of cancer.
8. Disinfectants and antiseptics.

A detailed study of the action of drugs on each organ is not necessary.

PRACTICAL **(50 Hours)**

The first six of the following experiments will be done by the students while the remaining will be demonstrated by the teacher.

1. Effect of K^+, Ca^{++}, acetylcholine and adrenaline on frog's heart.
2. Effect of acetylcholine on rectus abdominis muscle of frog and guinea pig ileum.
3. Effect on spasmogens and relaxants on rabbits intestine.
4. Effect of local anaesthetics on rabbit cornea.
5. Effect of mydriatics and miotics on rabbits eye.
6. To study the action of strychnine on frog.
7. Effect of digitalis on frog's heart.
8. Effect of hypnotics in mice.
9. Effect of convulsants and anticonvulsants in mice or rats.
10. Test for pyrogen.
11. Taming and hypnosis potentiating effect of chlorpromazine in mice/rats.
12. Effect of diphenhydramine in experimentally produced asthma in guinea pigs.

ANIMALS USED IN LABORATARIES

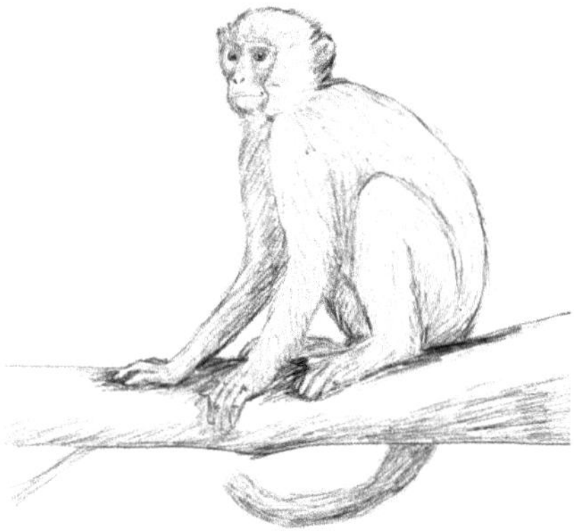

Monkey

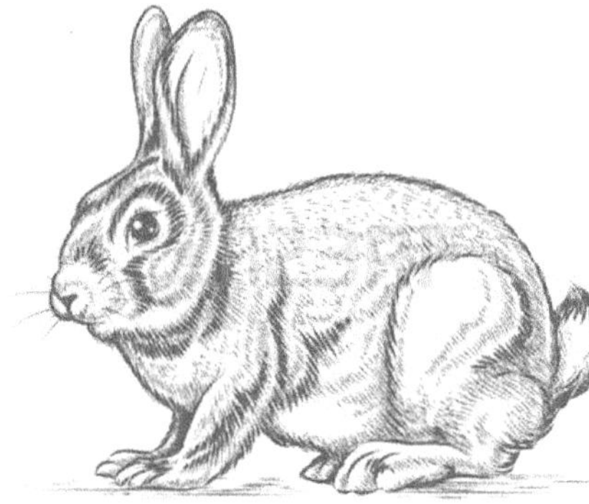

Rabbit

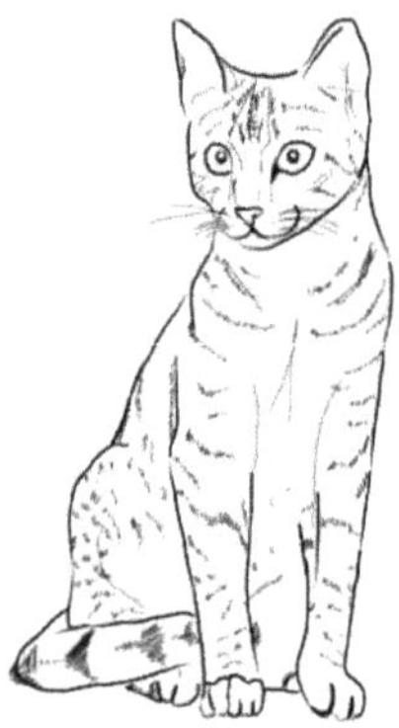

Cat

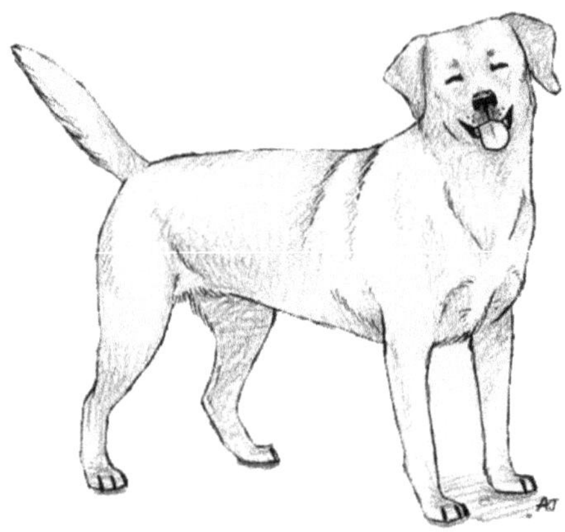

Dog

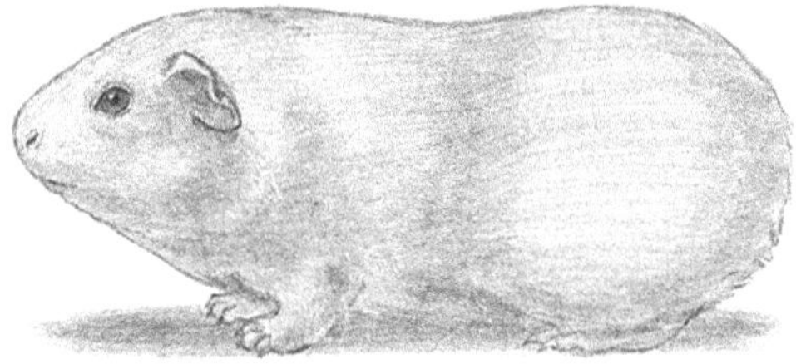

Guinean Pig

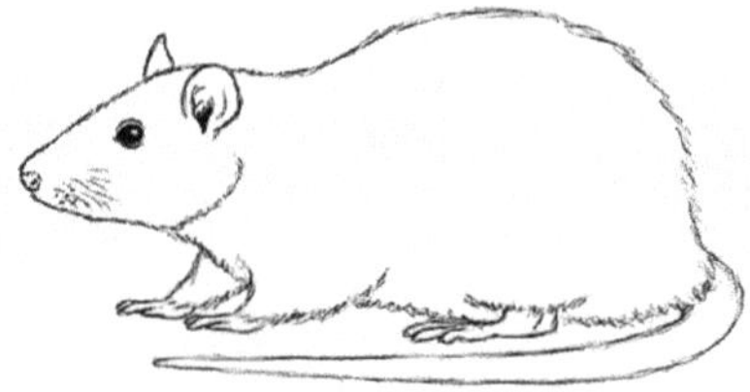

Albino Rat

SURGICAL INSTRUMENTS

Hemostatic Foreceps

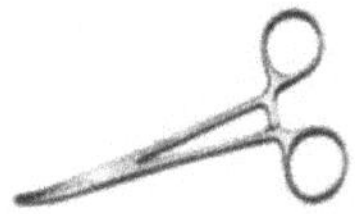
Artery Forceps

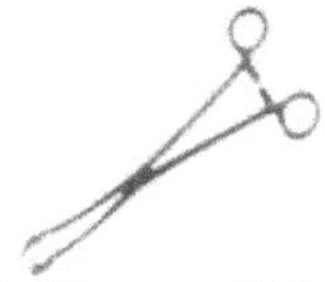
Konig Surgical Forceps with Teeth

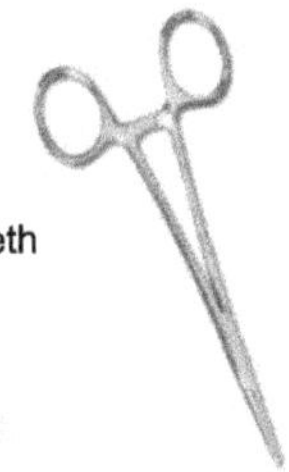
Halstead Mosquito Forceps

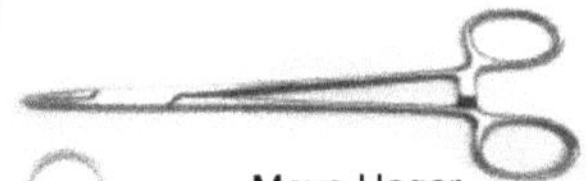
Mayo Hagar

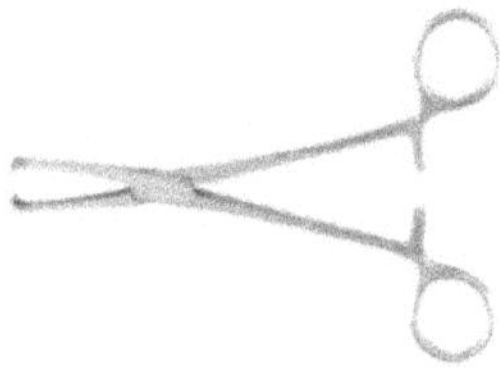
Allis Tissue Forceps 6"

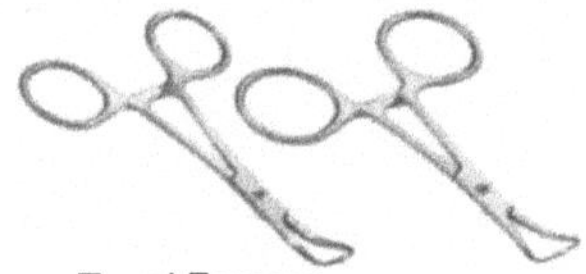
Towel Forceps

Surgical Scissors

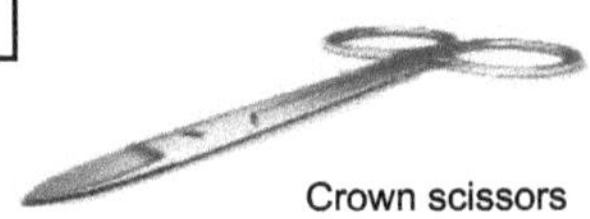
Crown scissors

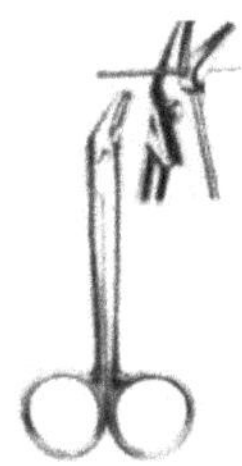
Roger wire scissors

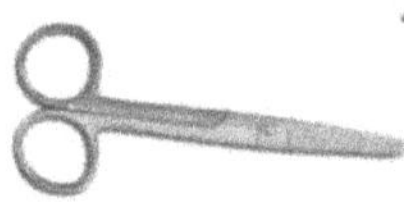
Dressing Scissors

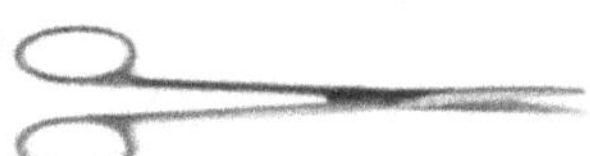
Curved Mayo Scissor-55in

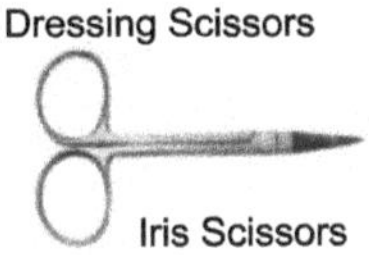
Iris Scissors

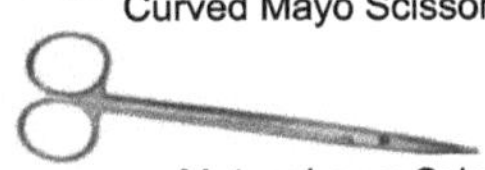
Metzenbaum Scissors

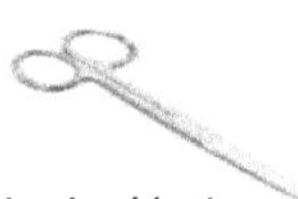
Nursing blunt

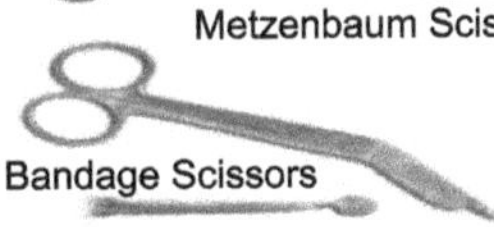
Bandage Scissors

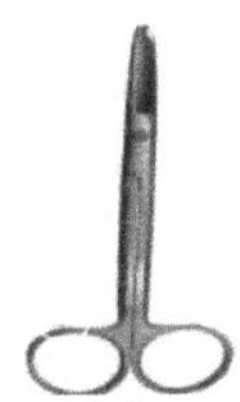
Stature ligature

Surgical Scissors

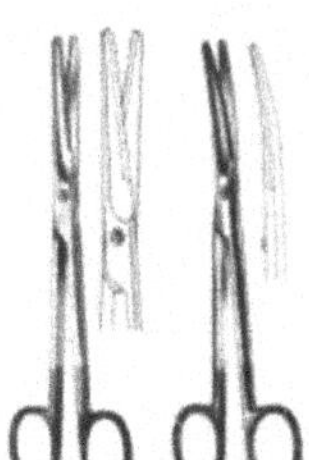
Mayo dissecting Tc.

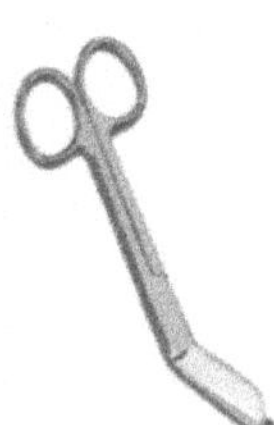
Lister Bandage

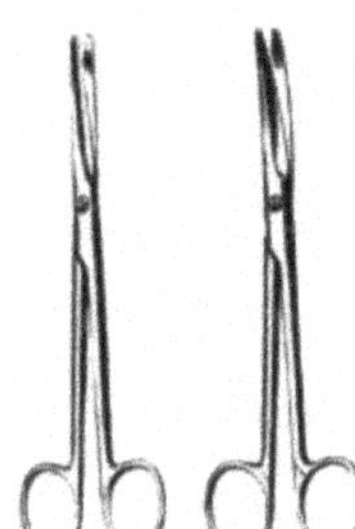
Mayo Dissecting Scissors

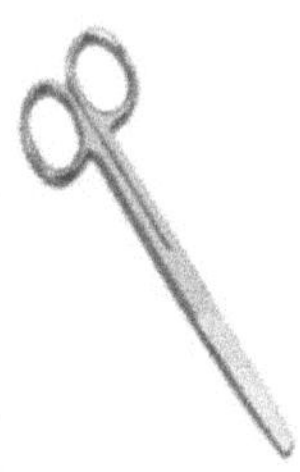
Dressing Scissors

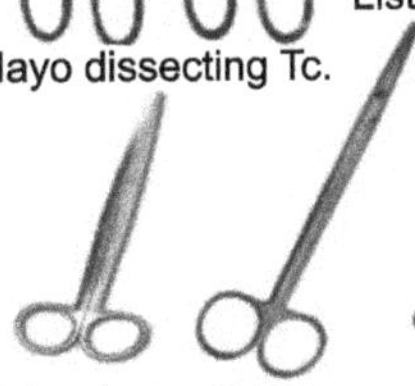
Metzenbaum Scissors

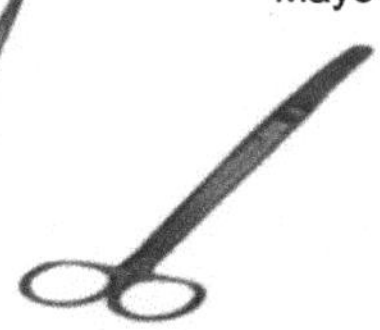
Uterine Scissors

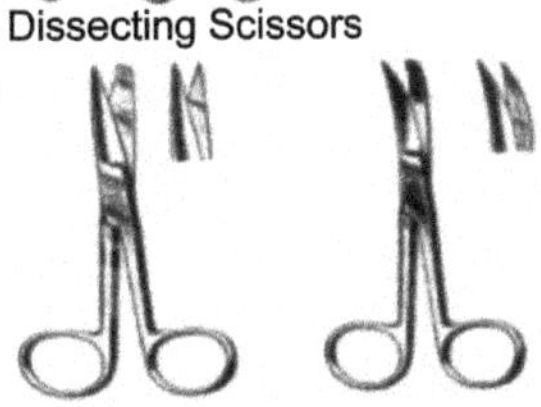
Deaver Scissors

COMMONLY USED LAB INSTRUMENTS

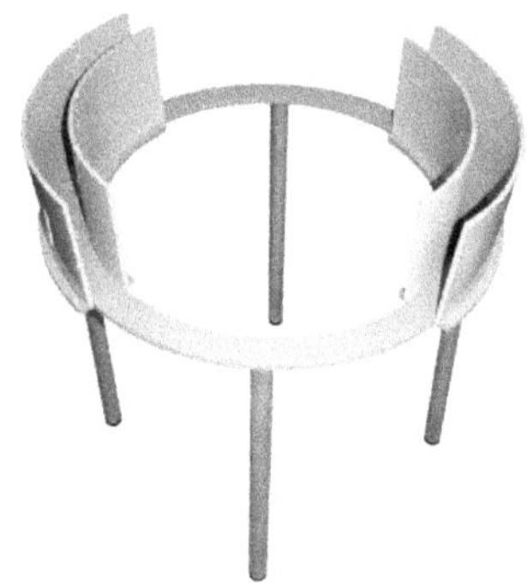

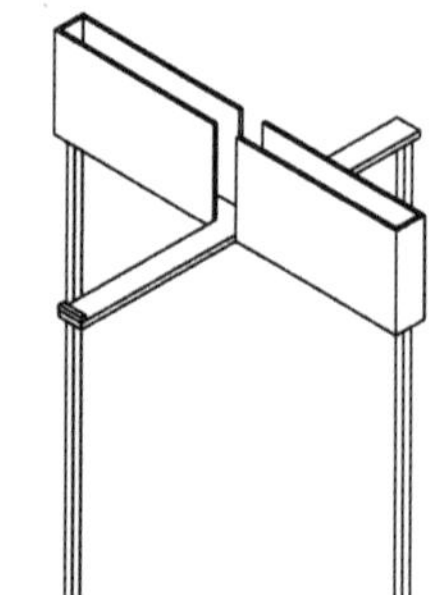

Isonetric view
Sacle : 1.4

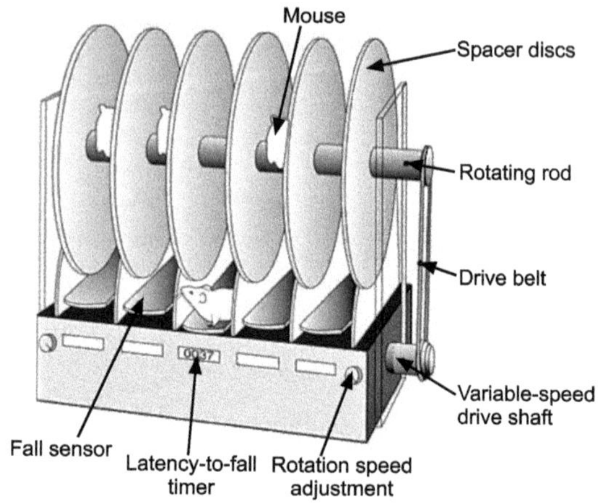

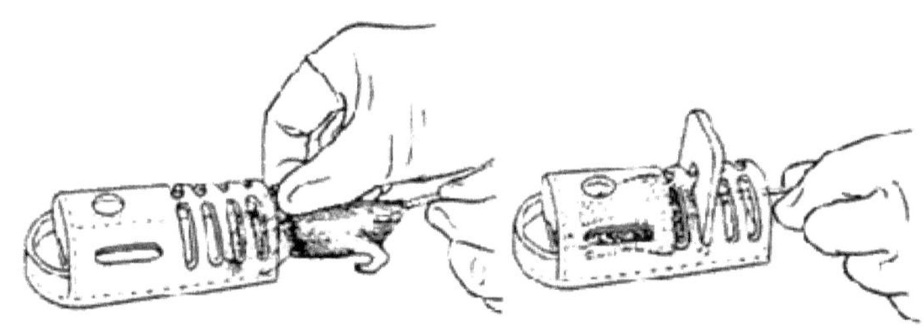

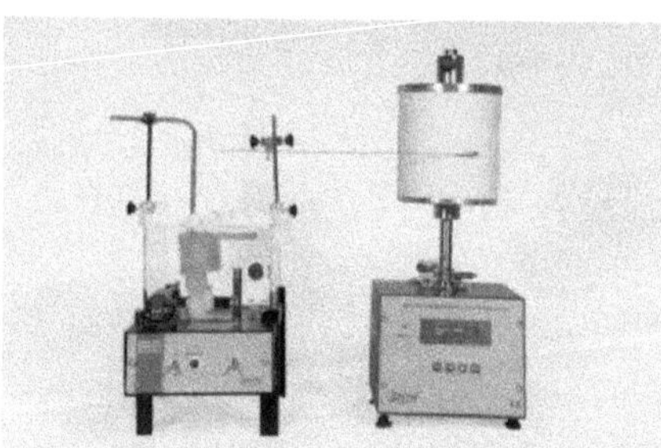

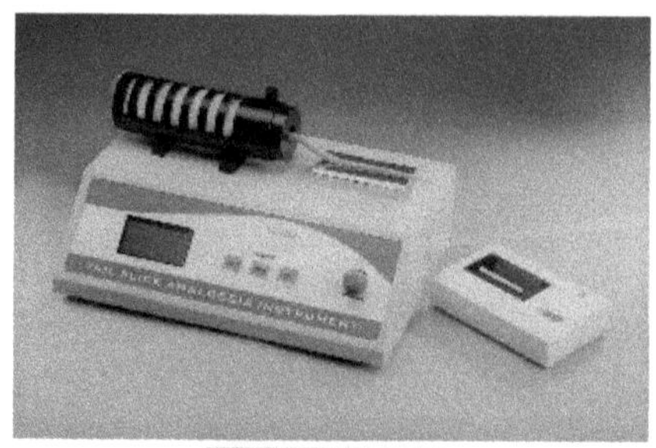

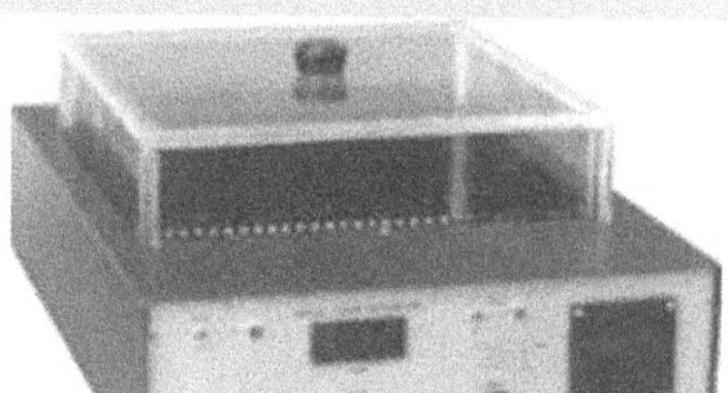

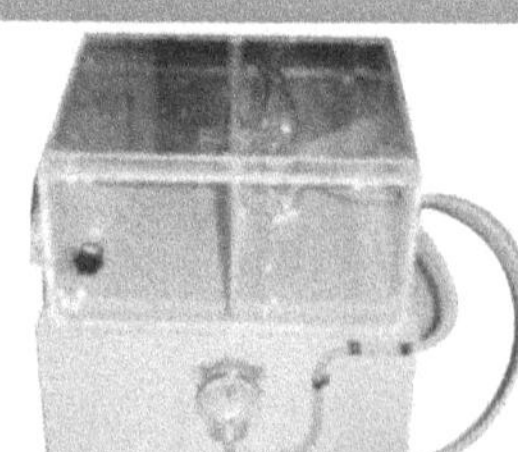

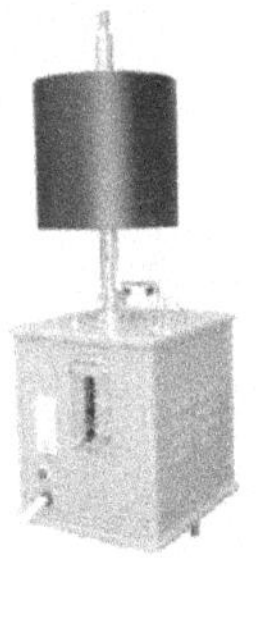

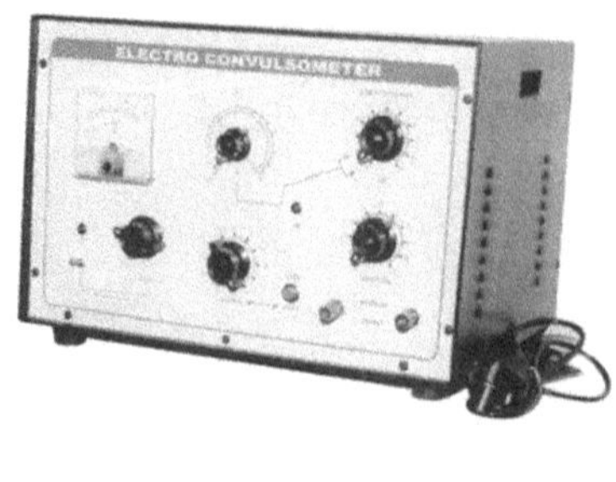

Index ...

Total marks obtained .... out of 150 **Sign of Subject Teacher**

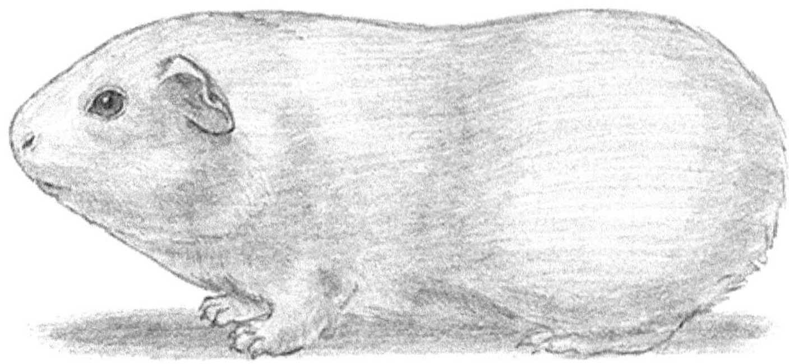

Guinea Pig

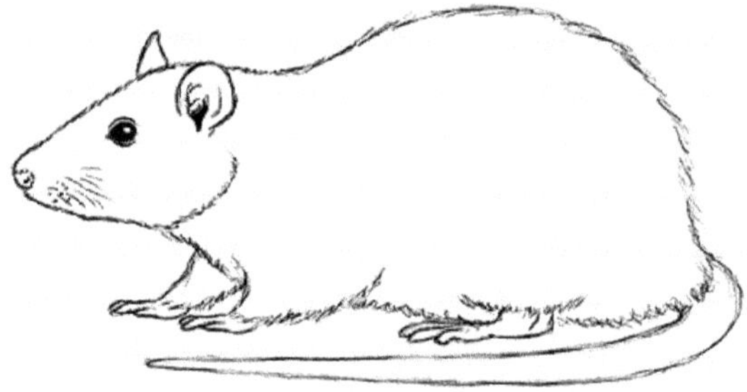

Albino Rat

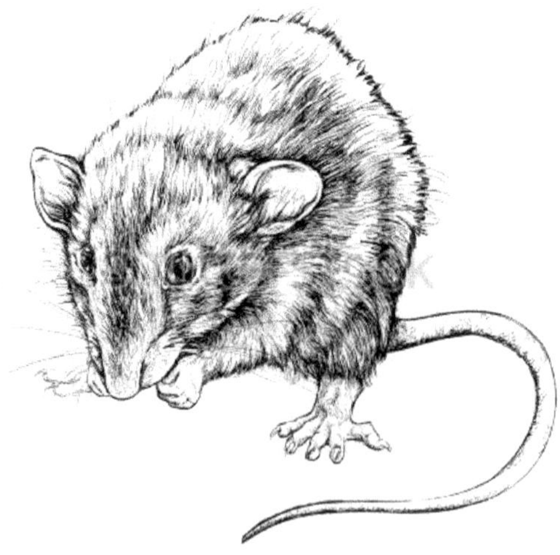

Albino Mouse

Figure: Commonly used Laboratory Animals

Date :__________ Marks : _______/10

EXPERIMENT NO. 1

- **Aim:** To study some commonly used laboratory animals.
- **Theory:** When a new drug molecule is discovered, we cannot simply test that drug molecule on human being. Before using it on humans, it should successfully pass the preclinical studies. Preclinical studies are studies which will be carried out on certain laboratory animals. Afterwards, the newly discovered drug, if it passes the preclinical studies, will be tested over the human population. Animals we use in our laboratory, generally are rats, mice, guinea pigs, frogs, monkeys, rabbits, dogs, etc. These animals should be chosen according to the demand of the experiment, financial conditions and convenience to store them. These animals are usually used because they have anatomical similarity with human beings. We suppose that drug will act similarly in these animals, as it is expected to work on our body itself. Following are some commonly used laboratory animals:
  1. **Guinea pig:** Guinea pigs (400-600 gm) are commonly used experimental animals. They are docile and easy to raise and maintain. They are highly sensitive to histamine. They are, therefore, used in experimental asthma to study bronchodilators. They are also used to study local anaesthetics and as models in experimental amoebiasis and cholera as they are sensitive to these micro-organisms. Guinea pig tissues (organs) such as ileum is the most common tissue preparation used to study spasmogens and antispasmodics. Guinea pig isolated heart and trachea are sensitive to histamine.
  2. **Albino rat:** White rats (wistar strain) are the commonest laboratory animals used in experimental pharmacology. Rats are easy to breed and maintain. Rats being small in size (200 gm), resemble human in several organ functions and nutrition, and sensitive to most of the drugs make them very useful experimental animals. However, they do not have vomiting centre and hence it is not possible to use them to study emetics. The various rat tissues such as colon, stomach, uterus, caecum and vas defences are used in testing various drugs. Beside these organs rat brain tissue is extensively employed in radio receptor ligand studies. There are several other species of rats which are used in laboratory.
  3. **Albino mouse:** White mice are the smallest laboratory animals used. Mice are also easy to breed and maintain. They are in small size (25-30 gm) and therefore, easy to handle. They are sensitive to most of the drugs used in experimental pharmacology. Mice are used extensively in toxicity study, bioassay of drugs, testing of analgesics, CNS active drugs etc. Mice brain tissues are also used in various biochemical estimations. There are several species of mice which can be used experimentally.

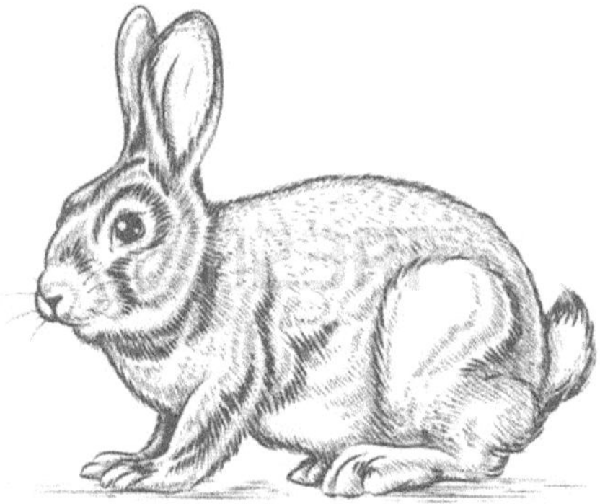

Rabbit

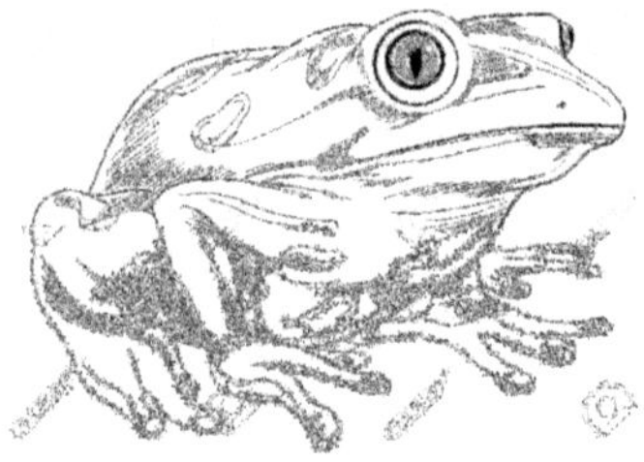

Frog

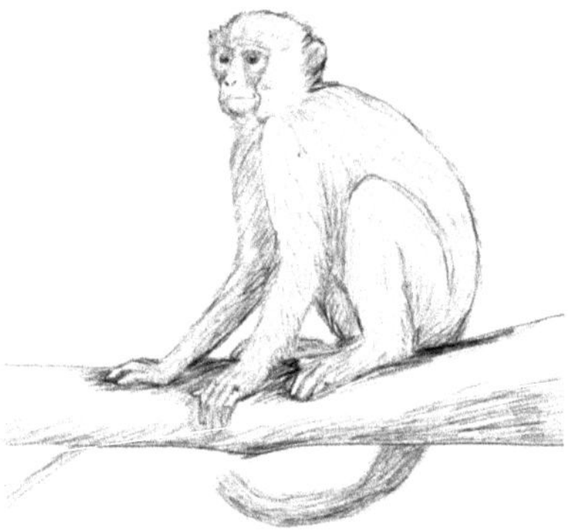

Monkey

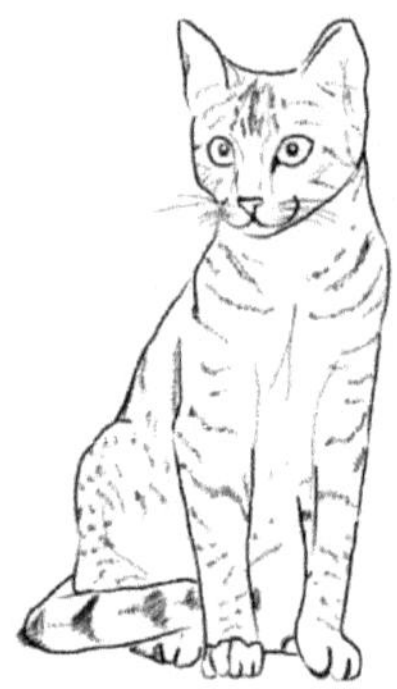

Cat

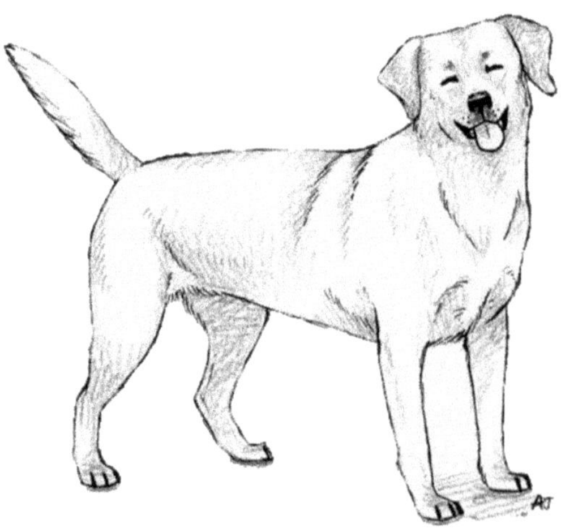

Dog

Figure: Commonly used laboratory animals

4. **Rabbit:** Domestic rabbits (2-3 kg) are generally used for pyrogen testing. Some of the tissues or organs from rabbits used are heart, aorta, duodenum, and ileum. One peculiar thing about rabbits is that they are resistant to the actions of atropine as they contain atropinesterase enzyme, the presence of which is genetically determined.
5. **Frog:** Frogs (150-250 gm) are also extensively used in experimental pharmacology. Isolated frog heart, rectus abdominis muscle preparation, study of muscle nerve preparation and ciliary movements are some of the organs of frog used. Frog is also used for the study of nerve block type of local anaesthetics. Frogs are inexpensive and easily available.
6. **Cat, Dog and Monkey:** Cats, dogs and monkeys are used for pharmacological investigation of drugs. Cats and dogs are commonly used to study blood pressure experiments. Monkeys are not used for routine pharmacological testing. Monkeys are quite expensive and are hard to maintain and breed.

- **Result:** The commonly used laboratory animals are studied.

VIVA VOCE QUESTIONS

Q.1 In which experiments we can use guinea pigs?

____

Q.2 Why do we prefer rodents in experimentations?

____

❖❖❖

Date :__________ Marks : ________/10

EXPERIMENT NO. 2

- **Aim:** To prepare physiological salt solution.
- **Theory:** The physiological salt solutions are used to keep isolated tissue or organ preparation surviving as long as the experiment is over. It is important to choose the particular type of solution in which tissue is known to survive. These physiological salt solutions are prepared carefully using analytical grade reagents and distilled water. The other precautions to be taken are adjusting the proper pH of the final solution and aeration with oxygen, mixture of oxygen and carbon dioxide (95% + 5%) or even bubbling with air. The physiological solution thus prepared should be clear and if it is turbid, then it is advised to prepare fresh solution before the start of the experiment. Some of the commonly used physiological salt solutions are mentioned below:
  1. ***Ringer, frog ringer and de Jalon solutions:*** These solutions do not contain any Mg or PO_4 ions. *Frog ringer* solution may also be prepared by adding 400 ml distilled water to one litre of *Ringer* solution. The composition of *de Jalon* is same as that of *ringer,* except it contains one forth the amount of $CaCl_2$ and half the amount of glucose.
  2. ***McEwen* solution** is sucrose in addition to glucose.
  3. ***Calcium-free ringer* solution** is identical to ringer solution, except that $CaCl_2$ is omitted.
  4. ***Calcium-free depolarizing ringer* solution** contains (mM) NaCl 94.0; KCl 60.0; $NaHCO_3$ 6.0; and dextrose 11.0.
  5. ***Zero-calcium depolarizing ringer* solution** has the same composition as *calcium-free depolarizing ringer* solution, except that it contains in addition EGTA 0.01.
  6. ***Potassium rich krebs* solution** is made by increasing KCl concentration upto 47.3 mM potassium at the expenses of an equivalent amount of NaCl.
  7. ***Low Na+ krebs* solution** is prepared by reducing NaCl to 38 mM and adding sucrose 150 mM to maintain the tonicity of the solution.
  8. ***Glucose free krebs* solution** is prepared by eliminating the glucose.
  9. ***Ringer solution*** is aerated with O_2 or air and used for mammalian isolated heart and other tissues; frog-ringer is used for frog heart and tissues.
  10. ***Tyrode* solution** is aerated with air, O_2 or 5% CO_2 in O_2 and used for mammalian smooth muscles.

  Krebs, modified Krebs-ringer's bicarbonate and McEwen solutions are aerated with 5% CO_2 in O_2 and used for mammalian isolated organs, especially for nerve responses.
- **Result:** The physiological salt solution is prepared.

VIVA VOCE QUESTIONS

Q.1 What is the difference between ringer and McEwen solution?

____

Q.2 What is the purpose of physiological salt solution?

____

❖❖❖

Date :__________ Marks : ________/10

EXPERIMENT NO. 3

- **Aim:** To study some commonly used isolated tissue preparations.
- **Theory:**

1. **Guinea pig ileum:** Healthy adult guinea pig is stunned by head blow, neck vessel cut, and the animal is bled out. Abdomen is opened through a midline incision, the ileocecal junction is exposed, the terminal ileum is cut after discarding 10 cm nearest to the ileocecal junction because of the presence of excitatory α-adrenoceptors near the ileocecal junction. The mesenteric attachment is cut as close to the gut as possible without injury for a distance of about 20 to 25 cm. The intestine is then cut across, and the lumen of the isolated piece is thoroughly cleaned by running warm salt solution repeatedly through the proximal opening, with the help of a 50 ml volumetric pipette. The clean strip of the intestine is then placed in fresh warm salt solution for a short period for acclimatization before being put up for the experiment. A small segment usually 4-6 cm in length is cut; at each end a thread is passed through the lumen with the help of sewing needle and is tied securely without occluding the lumen. One end of the segment is tied securely to the tissue holder or some other suitable contrivance and transferred to the organ bath. The second end of the tissue is tied to the frontal lever adjusted suitably for tension and magnification. Afterwards the practical can be started after two or three washings with physiological salt solution.
2. **Guinea pig tracheal chain:** Trachea is removed from freshly killed guinea pig and sectioned with a pair of scissors into 10 to 12 approximately equal size rings. Rings are kept moist in Ringer's solution while they are being tied in series by short loop of silk thread. The rings are oriented in such a way that the dorsal smooth muscle band is in a line. In an alternative but simpler method, the trachea is cut spirally or opened with a longitudinal cut along the mid-dorsal surface and a series of transverse cuts made successively from alternate sides so that they overlap one another but do not transect the preparation completely.
3. **Rat duodenum:** Proximal 3 cm of duodenum from freshly killed rat (150-250 gm) is dipped in salt solution at 4 to 6°C for two to three hours before use. It is suitable for identification of bradykinin that relaxes the preparation in very minute concentration, while substance P contracts it. The dose contact of drug in this preparation is usually 30 seconds at intervals of three to five minutes.
4. **Rat stomach:** The stomach from a freshly killed rat is dissected out and placed in the salt solution. The translucent fundus is cut along the pylorus leaving a thin band of the pyloric tissue attached to the fundus, and its content washed clean. The fundus is then cut open along the lesser curvature and spread on a cork mat soaked in salt solution. Alternative transverse cuts are made to preserve the

longitudinal muscle. The strip is then pulled out by cotton thread tied on each end and protrusions and fringes of pyloric tissue trimmed away to give a long clean thin strip for suspension in the bath.

5. **Rat uterus:** The uterus from the virgin rat (140-200 gm) is dissected out and the two horns are divided. One horn is suspended in the bath and the other horn is kept in salt solution at room temperature for later use, if needed. By using De Jalon solution the rhythmic contractions are abolished. The rat uterus is majorly used for the assay of oxytocin, 5-hydroxytryptamine and adrenaline.
6. **Rat anococcygeal muscle:** A male rat is killed by a blow to the head and bled. The abdomen is opened in the mid-line, the pelvis split, and the bladder and urethra removed taking care not to damage the ventral band of muscle lying ventral to the colon. The colon is then cut through at the pelvic brim, the pelvic portion pulled forward and the connective tissue cleaned until the anococcygeal muscles come into view. The two anococcygeal muscles in rat arise from the upper coccygeal vertebra behind the terminal colon, pass ventrocaudally to sweep round the lateral side of the colon, and unite in front of the colon a few mm from the anus to form a ventral band. The two muscles can be easily dissected out, and the extrinsic nerve that enters the deep surface of each muscle just short of the ventral band can be retained with the muscle for stimulation. The ventral band is cut through and each muscle is mounted in a 100 ml bath. The rat anococcygeal muscle is majorly used for the adrenergic neurons, muscarinic neurons and 5-HT receptors.
7. **Frog rectus muscle:** It is a voluntary muscle preparation producing slow contracture in response to acetylcholine. A pithed frog is laid on its back on the corkboard, the abdominal skin is cut away and the rectus muscle of one side is dissected from the pelvic girdle up to the pectoral girdle. The muscle is then pinned to the cork so as to keep it stretched to its normal length soaked in frog saline. A thread is sewn through each end and the muscle is then fixed in the bath, while the thread from the other end is fixed to a simple gimble lever. The preparation is suitable for the assay of acetylcholine as well as for curare like substances.

- **Result:** The commonly used isolated tissues are studied.

VIVA VOCE QUESTIONS

Q.1 Which drugs can we test on rat stomach preparations?

Q.2 Which drugs can we test on guinea pig ileum?

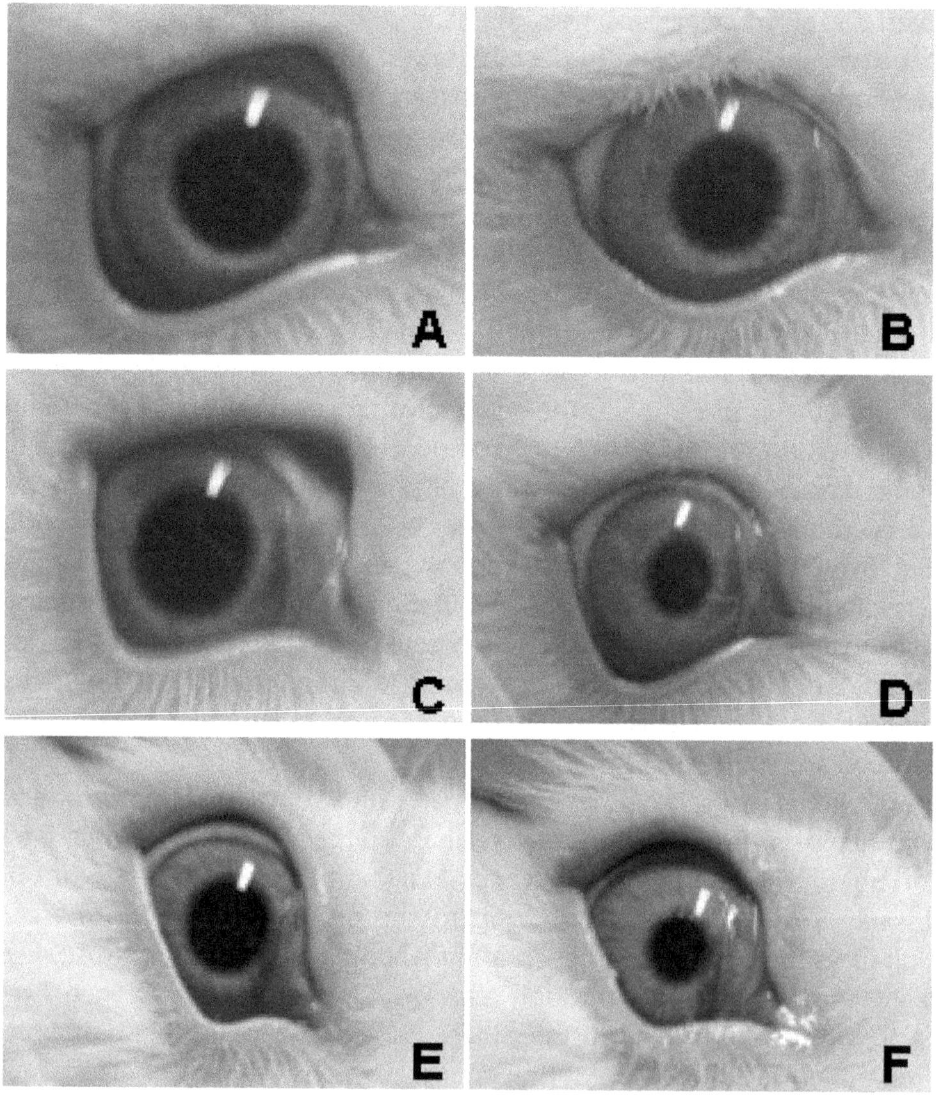

Figure: Mydriatic effect of atropine on rabbit eye

Date :__________ Marks : ________/10

EXPERIMENT NO. 4

- **Aim:** To study the mydriatic effect of atropine on rabbit eye.
- **Theory:** Local action of a large number of drugs in an eye can be achieved without systemic effect by the application of drugs as eye drops or eye ointments. Most of these drugs belong to antimicrobial, autonomic or local anaesthetic groups. The eye is supplied both by sympathetic and para-sympathetic nerves. The superior palpebral muscle and dilator pupillae (radial fibers) of the iris have sympathetic supply. The sphincter pupillae (circular fibers) of the iris have parasympathetic supply which exercises dominant control. The ciliary muscle is also supplied by para-sympathetic nerves and when it contracts, the ciliary body is moved inwards and forwards. Because of this the lens bulges forward and the eye is accommodated for near vision. The opposite effect is produced by the relaxation of ciliary muscle resulting in paralysis of accommodation. When the pupil dilates, the iris folds back near the opening of the canal of schlemn and the drainage of the aqueous humour is decreased thereby increasing the intraocular pressure. Constriction of the pupil by opposite action will increase drainage and reduce intraocular pressure.

  Topically applied drugs can affect the eye by changing the conjunctival congestion, pupillary size, light reflex, corneal sensitivity and intraocular pressure. However, the effect of the drugs on pupillary size, light reflex and corneal reflex can easily be studied by the students themselves.

  Physostigmine is a reversible cholinesterase inhibitor which increases the endogenous acetylcholine and stimulates the circular muscles of iris to produce pupillary constriction without producing loss of light reflex and corneal reflex. Ephedrine and phenylephrine stimulate the radial muscles of the iris to produce pupillary dilation without any effect on light reflex and corneal reflex. Atropine, an antimuscarinic agent, blocks the effect of endogenously released acetylcholine on the circular muscles of the iris and the muscles of the ciliary bed to produce mydriasis and spasm of accommodation leading to cycloplegia but without producing loss of corneal reflex.
- **Requirements:**

  Animals: Rabbits (2 kg),

  Drugs: Atropine, physostigmine.

  Equipments: Rabbit holder, torch light.

- **Procedure:**
  1. Place the rabbit in the rabbit box keeping the head outside.
  2. Observe size of the pupil in both eyes.
  3. Examine the effect of light reflex by holding the torch in front of the eye moving light beam to and fro.
  4. Examine the corneal reflex by touching a side of the cornea with a cotton piece.
  5. Instill a few drops of atropine solution in the conjunctiva (4-6 times) over the period of 8-10 minutes in the right eye of the rabbit. The left eye of the rabbit would serve as control. Instill normal saline in the left eye.
  6. Record the pupillary size, light reflex and corneal reflex after ten minutes of drug instillation and tabulate the observations.
  7. Repeat the experiment with physostigmine and ephedrine.

- **Result:** The mydriatic effect of atropine on rabbit eye is studied.

VIVA VOCE QUESTIONS

Q.1 What is the pharmacological action of physostigmine?

____

Q.2 What is the effect of physostigmine on eye?

____

❖❖❖

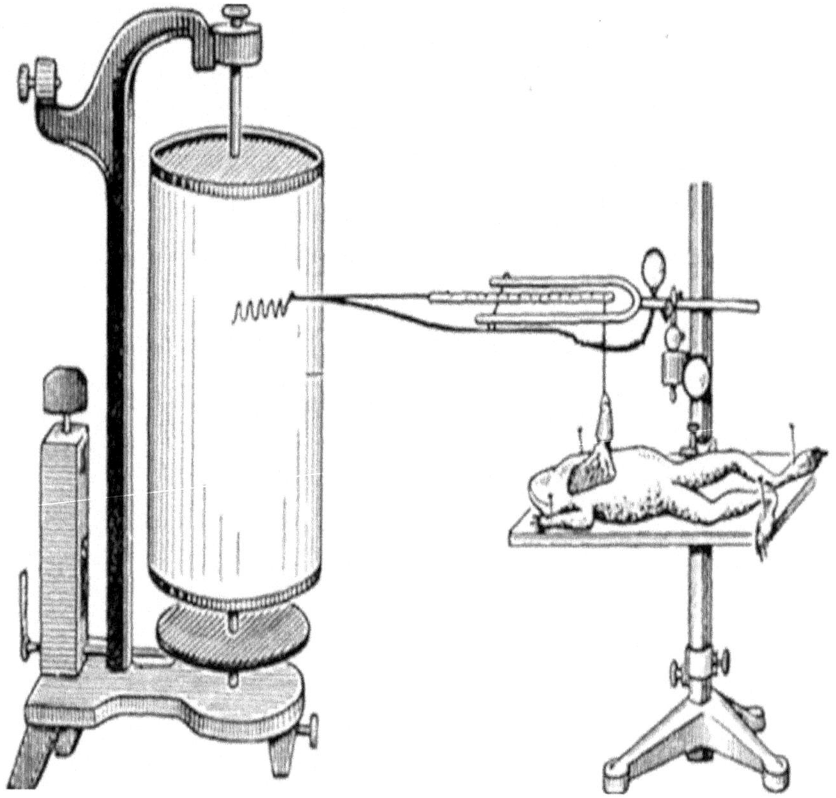

Figure: The effects of drugs on perfused frog heart.

Date :__________ Marks : ________/10

EXPERIMENT NO. 5

- **Aim:** To study the effects of drugs (inotropic and chronotropic actions) on perfused frog heart.
- **Theory:** Drugs may influence the rate (chronotrophy) and force (inotrophy) of contraction of the heart. An increase in the heart rate is called a positive chronotropic effect, while a negative chronotropic response is a decrease in heart rate. Similarly, an increase in the force of contraction is called a positive inotropic effect and a decrease in force of contraction is called negative inotropic effect. Sympathomimetic amines such as adrenaline and nor-adrenaline produce positive inotropic and positive chronotropic response. Whereas para-sympathomimetics such as acetylcholine produce negative inotropic and negative chronotropic response.
- **Requirements:**

  Animal: Frog

  Drugs: Adrenaline (stock solution 10 μg/ml),
  Nor-adrenaline (stock solution 10 μg/ml),
  Acetylcholine (stock solution 10 μg/ml),
  Calcium chloride (stock solution 10 μg/ml),
  Potassium chloride (stock solution 10 μg/ml).

  Physiological salt solution: Frog ringer.
- **Procedure:**
  1. Pith the frog and pin it to the frog board.
  2. Give a midline incision to the abdomen. Remove the pectoral girdle and expose the heart.
  3. Carefully remove the pericardium and put a few drops of frog ringer solution over the heart.
  4. Trace the inferior vena-cava, put a thread around it and give a small cut in order to insert the venous cannula which is in turn connected to a perfusion bottle containing frog ringer. Insert the cannula in the vein and tie the thread to assure the cannula in place.
  5. Give a small cut in one of the aortae for the perfusate to come out.
  6. Adjust a proper venous pressure of 2-4 cm by altering the height of perfusion bottle. The effective venous pressure is the height in cm from level of the venous cannula and the ringer level in the perfusion bottle. Use of the Marriott`s bottle helps in attaining the constant pressure. Start the perfusion by opening screw clamp attached to the tube.

7. Pass a thin pin hook through the tip of the ventricle, and with the help of a fine thread attached to the hook, tie it to the free limb of the universal lever, which is fixed to a stand. Adjust proper tension and magnification by altering the height of the lever. Record the normal contraction of the heart on the smoked drum.
8. Inject 0.1, 0.2, 0.5 and 1 ml of the stock solution of each drug in a sequential order and note the change in the rate and amplitude of contraction. Keep at least 5 minutes gap between the administration of each dose of the drug. The drug is administered by injecting the drug into the perfusion tube very close to the venous cannula. Take precaution to avoid any leakage of the drug from the tube, and the injection of air bubbles.
9. Label and fix the tracing with the fixing solution.

- **Result:** The effect of drugs (inotropic and chronotropic actions) on perfused frog heart is studied.

VIVA VOCE QUESTIONS

Q.1 Define chronotropic and inotropic effect.

____

Q.2 What will be the effect of adrenaline?

____

❖❖❖

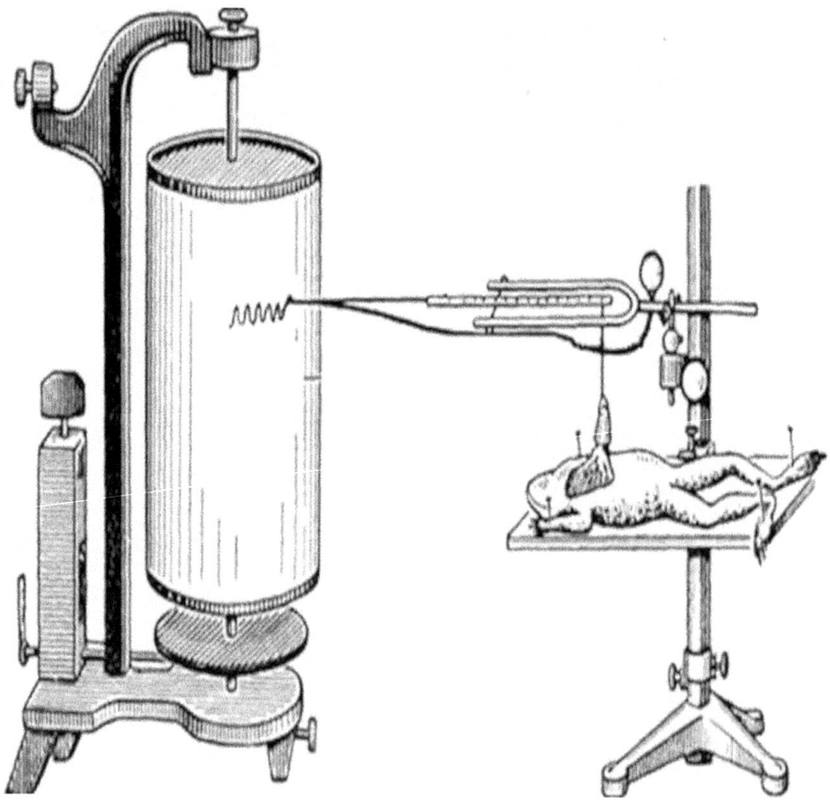

Figure: The effect digitalis on perfused frog heart

Date :__________ Marks : ________/10

EXPERIMENT NO. 6

- **Aim:** To record the effect of digitalis on frog's heart.
- **Theory:** The myocardial contraction of normal heart takes place according to Starling's law of heart. According to this law, force of systolic contraction is directly proportional to the fibre length in diastole. Since systolic contraction represents cardiac output and the fibre length in diastole indicated venous pressure, the law indicates that cardiac output is directly related to venous return or venous pressure during diastole. When the cardiac musculature fails to obey this relationship as in failing heart, there will be decrease in stroke volume (cardiac output), incomplete emptying of the ventricles during systole and enlargement of heart size due to residual blood in the heart at the end of systolic contraction. When the heart is in this state, *i.e.* inability to contract to physiological normal, it is said to be a hypodynamic heart. Experimentally hypodynamic heart can be produced by perfusing the heart with ringer containing less quantity of calcium as this bivalent ion is essential for myocardial contraction.
- **Requirements:**

  Animal: Frog.

  Drugs: Digitalis (digoxin stock solution 50 µg/ml).

  Physiological salt solution: Normal frog ringer and frog ringer containing $\frac{1}{4}^{th}$ $CaCl_2$.
- **Procedure:**
  1. Pith the frog and pin it to the frog board.
  2. Give a midline incision to the abdomen. Remove the pectoral girdle and expose the heart.
  3. Carefully remove the pericardium and put a few drops of frog ringer solution over the heart.
  4. Trace the inferior venacava, put a thread around it and give a small cut in order to insert the venous cannula which is in turn connected to a perfusion bottle containing frog ringer. Insert the cannula in the vein and tie the thread to assure the cannula in place.
  5. Give a small cut in one of the aortae for the perfusate to come out.
  6. Adjust a proper venous pressure of 2-4 cm by altering the height of perfusion bottle. The effective venous pressure is the height in centimetres from level of the

venous cannula and the ringer level in the perfusion bottle. Use of the Marriott's bottle helps in attaining the constant pressure. Start the perfusion by opening screw clamp attached to the tube.

7. Pass a thin pin hook through the tip of the ventricle, and with the help of a fine thread attached to the hook, tie it to the free limb of the universal lever, which is fixed to a stand. Adjust proper tension and magnification by altering the height of the lever. Record the normal contraction of the heart on the smoked drum.
8. Record the effect of 0.1, 0.2, 0.4 and 0.5 ml digoxin. Note the dose which gives adequate response.
9. Replace the perfusion fluid with modified ringer containing only $\frac{1}{4}^{th}$ the calcium chloride as compared to that of normal ringer. Note the change in pattern of recording of the heart.
10. When the heart is depressed markedly in presence of modified ringer, administer digoxin 0.1, 0.2, 0.4 and 0.5 ml. Note the change in contractility.
11. Fix the tracing and compare the responses of these drugs in normal and hypodynamic heart.

- **Result:** The effect of digitalis on frog's heart is studied.

VIVA VOCE QUESTIONS

Q.1 What are cardiac glycosides?

____

Q.2 What is the effect of Digitalis on heart rate?

____

❖❖❖

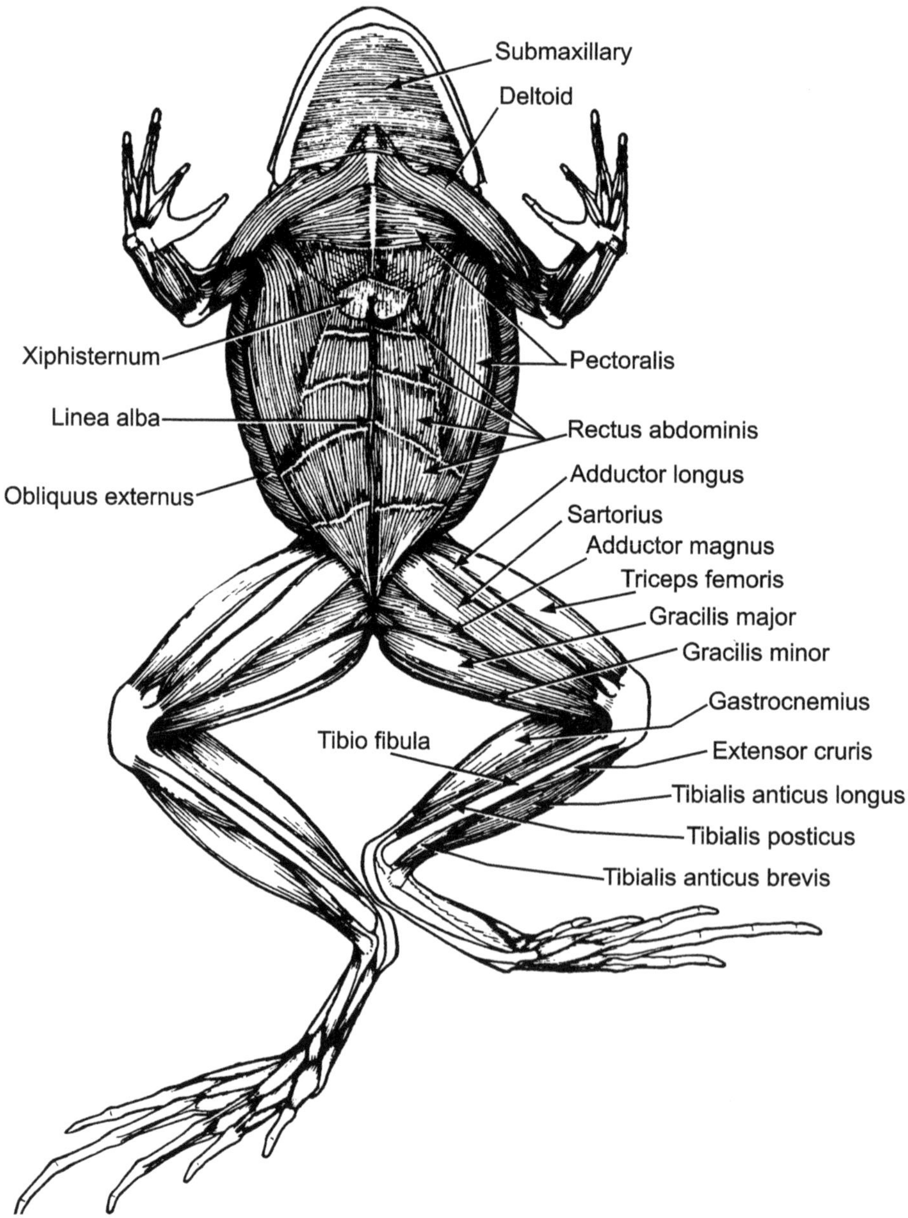

Figure: Rectus abdominis muscle of frog

Date :__________ Marks : ________/10

EXPERIMENT NO. 7

- **Aim:** To record the effect of acetylcholine on rectus abdominis muscle preparation of frog.
- **Theory:** Dose response curve (DRC) demonstrates graded responses to drugs or agonists where an increase in response is recorded with a subsequent increase in the dose or the concentration of the drug. The dose response curve is sigmoid or S-shaped. The first part (25% of graph) of the curve has poor discrimination between the doses, whereas the middle portion of the curve shows greater sensitivity to different concentrations, and the responses to increasing concentration are linearly differentiated. The last part of the curve shows the ceiling effect where no more increase in the response is seen with further increase in the dose.
- **Requirements:**
  Animal: Frog.
  Drugs: Acetylcholine stock solution (1 mg/ml).
  Physiological salt solution: Frog ringer.
- **Procedure:**
  1. Pith or stun the frog and lay it on its back on the frog-dissecting board. Pin the four limbs.
  2. Remove the skin on the abdomen and expose the rectus abdominis muscle.
  3. Cut and prepare two rectus muscle preparations from each frog. Tie a thread to the top and bottom of each muscle preparation before detaching the muscle from the body of the frog.
  4. Mount the preparation in up-right position in the organ bath containing frog ringer solution under a tension of 1 gm. There is no need of maintaining the bath temperature since it is an amphibian tissue preparation. Bubble the organ bath with air.
  5. Relax the tissue for 45 minutes, during which period wash the tissue with fresh quantum of ringer for at least four minutes.
  6. Record the concentration due to acetylcholine using either simple sideway or frontal writing lever. Ninety second contact time and a total 5 minutes time cycle may be used for proper recording of the responses.
  7. Record at least four responses to increasing dose of acetylcholine or till you get maximum response. The maximum response is achieved if one gets same of slightly less response with a higher concentration. Properly label the graph.
  8. Measure the height of response (mm) and draw a dose response curve graph.
- **Result:** The effect of acetylcholine on rectus abdominis muscle preparation of frog is studied.

VIVA VOCE QUESTIONS

Q.1 What are the pharmacological effects of acetylcholine?

____

Q.2 Why do we use frog ringer solution in this experiment?

____

❖❖❖

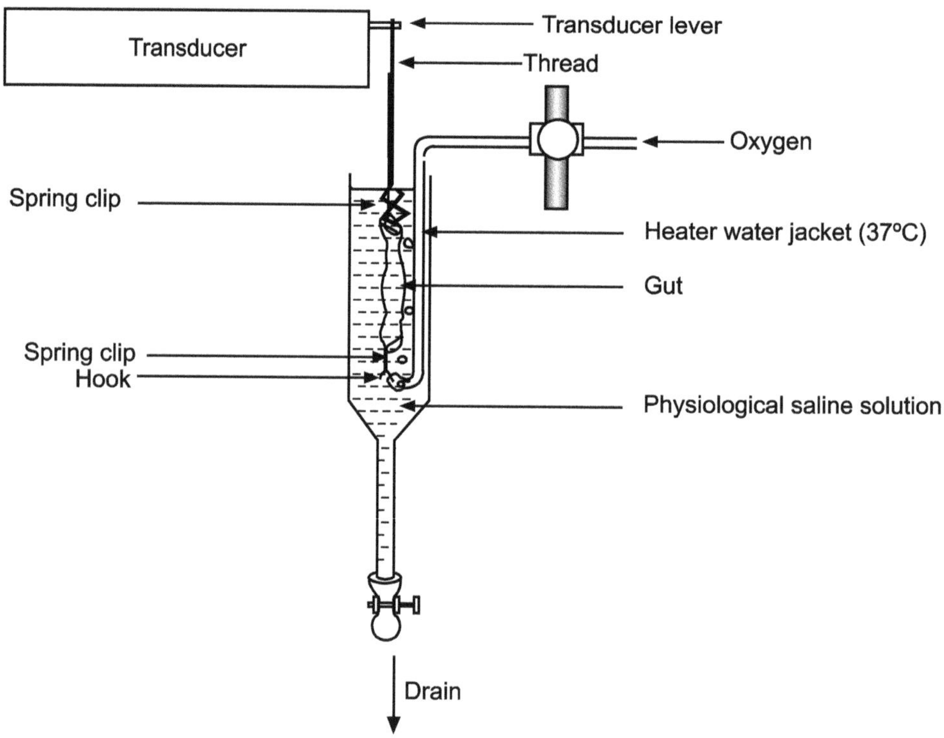

Figure: Organ Tube

Date :__________ Marks : ________/10

EXPERIMENT NO. 8

- **Aim:** To record the effect of acetylcholine on guinea pig ileum.
- **Theory:** Dose response curve (DRC) demonstrates graded responses to drugs or agonists where an increase in response is recorded with a subsequent increase in the dose or the concentration of the drug. The dose response curve is sigmoid or S-shaped. The first part (25% of graph) of the curve has poor discrimination between the doses, whereas the middle portion of the curve shows greater sensitivity to different concentrations, and the responses to increasing concentration are linearly differentiated. The last part of the curve shows the ceiling effect where no more increase in the response is seen with further increase in the dose.
- **Requirements:**
  Animals: Guinea pig (400-600 gm, overnight fasted).
  Drugs: Acetylcholine stock solution 01 mg/ml.
  Physiological Salt Solution: Tyrode.
- **Procedure:**
  1. The guinea pig is sacrificed by a blow on the head and carotid bleeding.
  2. Cut open the abdomen and lift the caecum to trace the ileocecal junction. Cut and remove a few centimetre long of the ileal portion and immediately place it in the watch glass containing Tyrode solution. Trim the mesentery and with gentle care clean the content of the ileum by pushing the Tyrode solution into the lumen of the ileum. Utmost care should be taken to avoid any damage to the gut muscle. Cut the lumen into small segments of 2-3 cm.
  3. Take one piece of ileum of 2-3 cm long and tie the thread to top and the bottom ends without closing the lumen, and mount the tissue in the organ bath containing Tyrode solution maintained at 32-35°C and bubbled with O_2 or air. A tension of 0.5 g is applied and the tissue is allowed to equilibrate for 30 min before adding drugs to the organ bath.
  4. Record concentration dependent response due to acetylcholine using frontal lever. Contact times of 30 seconds and 5 minutes time cycle are kept for proper recording of the response.
  5. Record at least 4 concentration dependent responses or maximum responses due to acetylcholine.
  6. Measure the length of the responses in mm.
  7. Draw a dose response curve using obtained values.
- **Result:** The effect of acetylcholine on guinea pig ileum is studied.

VIVA VOCE QUESTIONS

Q.1 Which PSS we had used in this experiment?

____

Q.2 Name the parts of small intestine?

____

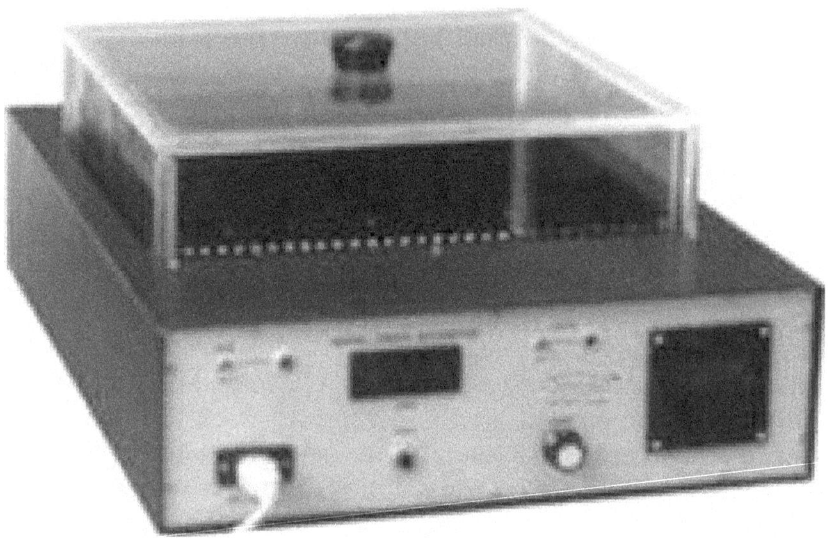

Figure: Actophotometer

Date :___________ Marks : ________/10

EXPERIMENT NO. 9

- **Aim:** To study the hypnotic effect of chlorpromazine in mice using actophotometer.
- **Theory:** Most of the central nervous system acting drugs influence the locomotor activities in man and animals. The CNS depressant drugs such as barbiturates and alcohol reduce the motor activity, while the stimulants such as caffeine and amphetamines increase the activity. In other words, locomotor activity can be an index of wakefulness of mental activity.

  The locomotor activity can be easily measured using an actophotometer which operates on photoelectric cells which are connected in circuit with a counter. When the beam of light falling on the photocell is cut off by the animal, a count is recorded. An actophotometer could have either circular or squared arena in which the animal moves. Both rats and mice may be used for testing in this experiment.
- **Requirements:**

  Animals: Mice (20-25 gm).

  Drugs: Chlorpromazine hydrochloride (dose 3 mg/kg, i.p.; make a stock solution containing 0.3 mg/ml of the drug and inject 1 ml/100 g body weight of mouse).

  Equipment: Actophotometer.
- **Procedure:**
  1. Weigh the animals and number them.
  2. Turn on the equipment (check and make sure that all the photo-cells are working for accurate recording) and place individually each mouse in the activity cage for 10 minutes. Note the basal activity score of all the animals.
  3. Inject chlorpromazine (1 ml/100 g) and after 30 minutes, retest each mouse for activity scores for 10 minutes. Note the difference in the activity, before and after the chlorpromazine.
  4. Calculate per cent decrease in motor activity.
- **Result:** The hypnotic effect of chlorpromazine in mice using actophotometer is studied.

VIVA VOCE QUESTIONS

Q.1 What dose of chlorpromazine we had used in this experiment?

____

Q.2 What is the principle of actophotometer?

____

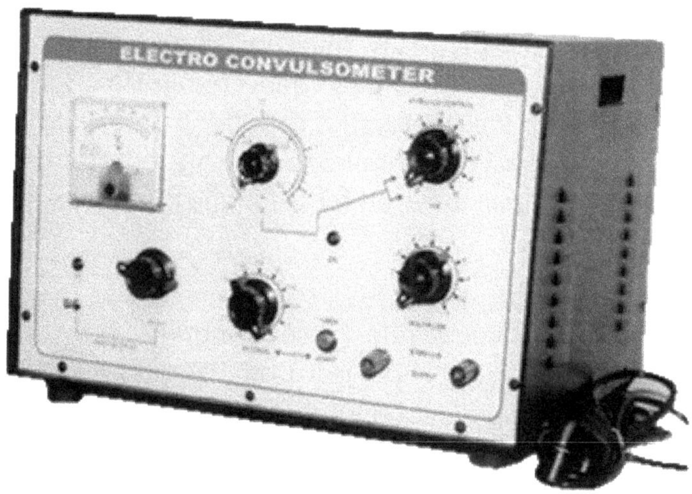

Figure: Convulsometer

Date :__________ Marks : ________/10

EXPERIMENT NO. 10

- **Aim:** To study anticonvulsant activity of phenytoin against electro-shock induced convulsions in rats.
- **Theory:** Different types of epilepsies, *i.e.* grand mal, petit mal or psychomotor type, can be studied in laboratory animals. The maximal electro-shock induced convulsions in animals represent grand mal type of epilepsy. Similarly, chemo-convulsions due to pentylenetetrazol which produce clonic type convulsions resemble petit mal type of epilepsy. These are the two procedures used to study convulsions and to test anticonvulsant drugs in laboratory animals.

  The MES-convulsions electroshock is applied through the corneal electrodes. Through optic stimulation cortical excitation is produced. The MES-convulsions are divided into five phases such as (a) tonic flexion, (b) tonic extensor, (c) clonic convulsion, (d) stupor and (e) recovery or death. A substance is known to possess anticonvulsant property if it reduces or abolishes the extensor phase of MES-convulsions. This procedure may be used to produce convulsion both in rats and mice.
- **Requirements:**

  Animals: Rats (150-200 gm).

  Drugs: Phenytoin (dose 25 mg/kg; prepare a stock solution containing 5 mg/ml of the drug and inject 0.5 ml/100 g body weight of animal).

  Equipment: Electro-convulsometer, corneal electrode, stop watch.
- **Procedure:**
  1. Weigh and number the animals. Divide them into two groups each consisting of 4-5 rats. One group is used as control group and the other for drug treatment.
  2. Hold the animal properly, place corneal electrodes on the cornea and apply prescribed current. Note different stages of convulsions.
  3. Note the time spent by animal in each phase of convulsion. Repeat with other animals of control group.
  4. Inject phenytoin intraperitoneally to a group of 4-5 rats. Wait for 30 minutes and subject the animals to electro-convulsions.
  5. Note the reduction in time of tonic extensor phase of MES-convulsions.
- **Result:** The anticonvulsant activity of phenytoin against electro-shock induced convulsions in rats is studied.

VIVA VOCE QUESTIONS

Q.1 In which disease we use phenytoin?

____

Q.2 Which instrument we had used in this experiment?

____

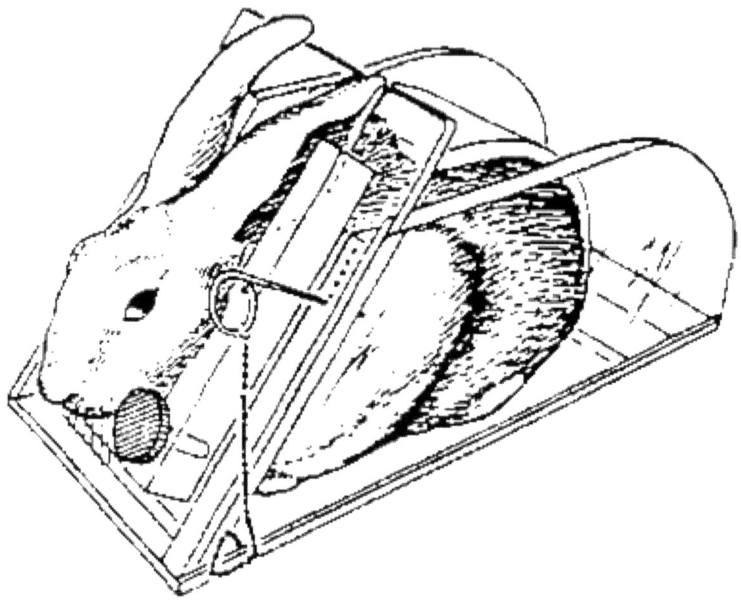

Figure: Sham Test for Pyrogen

Date :___________ Marks : ________/10

EXPERIMENT NO. 11

- **Aim:** To carry out test for presence of pyrogen (Sham Test).
- **Theory:** Rabbits are very sensitive to pyrogen. Therefore, when pyrogen containing solution is given intravenously, it produces a rise in body temperature within 3 hours. If the parenteral solution is sterile, it does not produce any rise in temperature. The sample which produces a rise of 24°C is considered to be pyrogenic and discarded.
- **Requirements:**

  Animal: Rabbits having body weight not less than 1.5 kg.

  Equipment: Rabbit restrainer, Tele-thermometer, disposable needles and syringes.
- **Procedure:**
  1. Select healthy rabbits and keep them in the animal room maintained at a temperature of 22 ± 2°C for 3 weeks period. Proper feed and water should be provided.
  2. Perform Sham Test in an air-conditioned room (i.e. inject pyrogen free solution (10 ml/kg, i.v.) and record the rectal temperature using tele-thermometer for 3 hours at 30 minutes interval.).
  3. Give three days' rest to the animals.
  4. Record the initial temperature for each animal at 30 minutes interval for a period of 90 minutes. Do not select rabbits having initial temperature above 39.8 °C and below 38°C.
  5. Administer the preparation to be tested for pyrogen by intravenous route (10 ml/kg) through the marginal ear vein.
  6. Record the temperature for each rabbit at 30 minutes interval for a period of 3 hours.
  7. Find out the difference between initial and final temperature for each rabbit. This is taken to be its response.
- **Result:** The test for presence of pyrogen (Sham Test) is studied.

VIVA VOCE QUESTIONS

Q.1 Why do we use rabbits in this experiment?

____

Q.2 What is the effect of pyrogen on body?

____

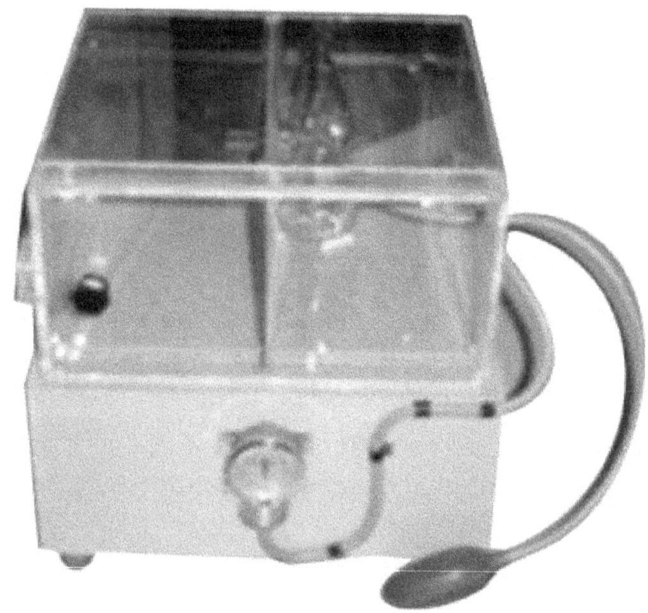

Figure: Histamine Chamber

Date :__________ Marks : ________/10

EXPERIMENT NO. 12

- **Aim:** To record the effect of diphenhydramine in experimentally produced asthma in guinea pigs.
- **Theory:** Asthma is characterised by bronchospasm and difficulty in breathing. These effects are mediated by autocoids like histamine, leukotrienes, platelet activating factor, serotonin, kinin, etc. Guinea pig is very sensitive to histamine. When guinea pig is exposed to histamine vapours, it exhibits bronchospasm, difficulty in breathing and convulsions. These effects of histamine are mediated through the action of histamine H1 receptor blocker. Therefore, diphenhydramine prevents the bronchospasm induced by histamine.
- **Requirements:**

  Animals: Guinea pigs.

  Apparatus: Histo-meter, Stop watch, Disposable needle and syringe.

  Drugs: Normal saline, diphenhydramine (5 mg/ml), histamine diphosphate (30 μg/ml).
- **Procedure:**
  1. Select 4 guinea pigs having body weight 250-300 gm.
  2. Fast the guinea pigs for 12 hours before experiment.
  3. Divide the animals in two equal groups, weigh them and mark them.
  4. Give normal saline (1 ml/kg, *i.p.*) to group I and diphenhydramine (5 mg/kg, *s.c.*) to group II.
  5. After one hour, place each guinea pig in histamine chamber and replace the cover.
  6. With the help of the compressor, spray a finely atomised mist of histamine diphosphate (30 μg/ ml) from nebuliser in both compartments.
  7. Using the stopwatch record the time of histamine administration.
  8. Observe the sign of respiratory distress (difficulty and cessation of breathing and convulsions) and the animals falling at its side.
  9. Record the observations.
- **Result:** The effect of diphenhydramine in experimentally produced asthma in guinea pigs is studied.

VIVA VOCE QUESTIONS

Q.1 What is the effect of diphenhydramine?

____

Q.2 Why do we use guinea pig in this experiment?

____

❖❖❖

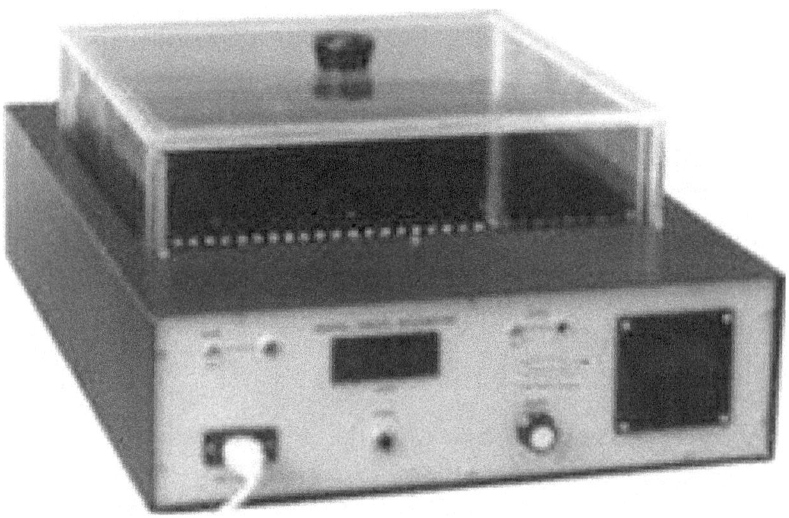

Figure: Actophotometer for Hypnotics Test

Date :__________ Marks : ________/10

EXPERIMENT NO. 13

- **Aim:** To record the effects of various hypnotics in mice.
- **Theory:** Sedative drugs supress the responsiveness to the constant stimulation. They decrease the spontaneous motor activities. Hypnotics are drugs which induce sleep resembling natural sleep. Hypnotics in higher dose produce anaesthesia.

  Benzodiazepines and barbiturates both are potent hypnotic agents. They bind to $GABA_A$ receptor and hence reduce the motor activities. Barbiturates also inhibit the excitatory AMPA- glutamate receptor which leads to the decreased motor functions. Thus they both act as central nervous system depressants.
- **Requirements:**

  Animals: Albino mice weighing 25-30 gm.

  Apparatus: Actophotometer, stopwatch, needles and syringes.

  Drugs: Normal saline, phenobarbitone 3 mg/ml, phenobarbitone 4 mg/ml, nitrazepam 0.5 mg/ml.
- **Procedure:**
  1. Select 20 albino mice.
  2. Fast them for 12 hours before experiment.
  3. Divide them into four groups each consisting of five animals, mark them and keep them in different cages.
  4. Put each group of mice into an actophotometer and record the motor activity for 30 minutes.
  5. After 30 minutes remove each group of animals from actophotometer.
  6. Administer normal saline to Group I, phenobarbitone sodium 30 mg/kg to Group II, Phenobarbitone 40 mg/kg to Group III, Nitrazepam 5 mg/kg to Group IV orally.
  7. Record the observations for each group.

- **Result:** The effects of various hypnotics in mice are studied.

VIVA VOCE QUESTIONS

Q.1 What the mechanism of action of barbiturates?

____

Q.2 What is the difference between sedatives and hypnotics?

____

❖❖❖

Date :__________ Marks : ________/10

EXPERIMENT NO. 14

- **Aim:** To study the effect of spasmogens and relaxants on rabbit intestine.
- **Theory:** Rabbit intestine is a smooth muscle which shows regular pendular movement (i.e. continuous contraction and relaxation). Therefore, to study the effect of drugs on intestinal movement rabbit intestine is an ideal preparation. Rabbit intestine is supplied by autonomic nervous system. Rabbit intestine contains muscarinic receptors and adrenergic receptors. Muscarinic receptor agonist like acetylcholine produces contraction of rabbit intestine and physostigmine increases the spasm and pendular movements. The above muscarinic actions and effects can be blocked by muscarinic blockers.

  Adrenaline acts on alpha and beta receptors and exhibits inhibitory effects on pendular movement. The action of adrenaline is blocked by adrenoceptor blockers like alpha receptor blockers and beta receptor blockers.
- **Requirements:**

  Animals: Rabbits weighing 1 to 1.5 kg.

  Physiological salt solution: Tyrode solution.

  Drugs: Acetylcholine chloride 20 μg/ml, Physostigmine sulphate 10 μg/ml, Atropine 4 μg/ml, adrenaline hydrogen sulphate 20 μg/ml and propranolol hydrochloride 100 μg/ml.
- **Apparatus:** Kymograph, student organ bath assembly, tuberculine syringe, needle (26 no. gauge), scissors, forceps.
- **Procedure:**
  1. Fast the rabbit for 12 hours before experiment.
  2. Set the assembly for rabbit intestine experiment, prepare the Tyrode solution.
  3. Kill the rabbit by giving a blow on its head and cutting the carotid artery.
  4. Open the abdominal region and identify the intestine.
  5. Remove a length of intestine (approximately 3-4 cm) and using surgical suturing needle tie a thread at each end, taking care to see that the lumen of the intestine remained open.
  6. Tie one end of the thread to the hook of the aeration tube and the other to a frontal writing lever.
  7. Stabilise the tissue for 30 minutes period.
  8. Aerate the rabbit intestine in the inner organ bath with a mixture of oxygen (95 %) and carbon dioxide (5 %).

9. Record the normal pendular movement of the rabbit intestine on the drum for 30 seconds. At the end of 30 seconds add 0.1 ml of acetylcholine into the inner organ bath and record the spasmogenic effect of the drug for 30 seconds. After recording the response for 30 seconds switch off the kymograph. Immediately open the outlet of the inner organ bath and remove the Tyrode solution present in the inner organ bath. Again fill the inner organ bath with fresh Tyrode solution and keep it for 60 seconds. Repeat the washing procedure 3-4 times or till the writing point of frontal lever comes to the normal pendular movement base line.
10. Then record the response of 0.1 ml physostigmine solution. Give 3-4 washings for recovery.
11. Record the response of 0.1 ml adrenaline solution. Give 3-4 washings for recovery.
12. Add 0.1 ml of atropine sulphate solution into the inner organ bath, allow it to act for 60 seconds, then record the response of acetylcholine in the presence of atropine sulphate. Give 3-4 washings for the recovery.
13. Add 0.1 ml of atropine sulphate solution into the inner organ bath, allow it to act for 60 seconds, then record the response physostigmine solution in presence of atropine sulphate. Give 3-4 washings for recovery.
14. Add 0.1 ml of propranolol solution into the inner organ bath, allow it to act for 60 seconds, then record the response of adrenaline solution in the presence of propranolol. Give 3-4 washings for recovery.

- **Result:** The effect of spasmogens and relaxants on rabbit intestine is studied.

VIVA VOCE QUESTIONS

Q.1 What are spasmogens?

____

Q.2 What is the effect of atropine on intestine?

____

❖❖❖

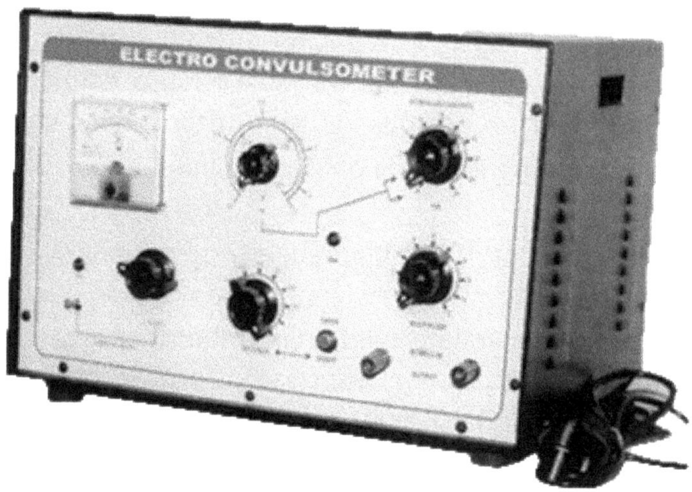

Figure: Convulsometer

Date :___________ Marks : ________/10

EXPERIMENT NO. 15

- **Aim:** To study the central nervous system stimulant and convulsant effect of Strychnine hydrochloride in frog.
- **Theory:** Strychnine is a powerful central nervous system stimulant and convulsant. The main site of action of strychnine is spinal cord. Glycine is an inhibitory neurotransmitter present in the spinal cord. Strychnine antagonises the action of glycine and produces convulsions.
- **Requirements:**

  Animal: Frogs.

  Drugs: Normal saline, Strychnine hydrochloride 4 mg/ml.
- **Procedure:**
  1. Weigh six frogs and divide them into two groups each comprising of three frogs. Keep them in a plastic cage.
  2. Administer normal saline (1 ml/kg body weight) to group I by subcutaneous injection.
  3. Administer strychnine hydrochloride (4 mg/kg body weight) subcutaneously to group II and note time of administration of strychnine hydrochloride.
  4. Observe the onset, severity and duration of hyperflex activity and convulsion produced in each frog.
  5. Record the observations.
- **Result:** The central nervous system stimulant and convulsant effect of Strychnine hydrochloride in frog is studied.

VIVA VOCE QUESTIONS

Q.1 What is the pharmacological significance of strychnine?

____

Q.2 Why are we using two groups?

____

❖❖❖

NOTES

NOTES

www.ingramcontent.com/pod-product-compliance
Ingram Content Group UK Ltd.
Pitfield, Milton Keynes, MK11 3LW, UK
UKHW051318160826
14477UKWH00027B/691